The information  contained in this eBook is for general information purposes only. While we try to keep the information up-to-date and correct, there are no representations or warranties, express or implied, about the completeness, accuracy, reliability, suitability or availability with respect to the information, products, services, or related graphics contained in this eBook for any purpose. Any use of this information is at your own risk. The methods describe within this book are the author's personal thoughts. They are not intended to be a definitive set of instructions for this project. You may discover there are other methods and materials to accomplish the same end result. This book is not intended to be a substitute for the medical advice of a licensed physician. The reader should consult with their doctor in any matters relating to his/her health.

© 2018 Claudia J. Caldwell | Florian Funk All rights reserved.

This book or parts thereof may not be reproduced in any form, stored in any retrieval system, or transmitted in any form by any means—electronic, mechanical, photocopy, recording, or otherwise—without prior written permission of the publisher, except as provided by United States of America copyright law. For permission requests, write to the publisher, at "Attention: Permissions Coordinator," at the address below.

info@cj-caldwell.com

Keto Spirit:
Defy Aging and Weight Gain with the Diet of Your Dreams

Discover the Diet That Lets You Beat Off the Pounds, Fight Weight-Related Illness, and Feel Young Again!

By

Claudia J. Caldwell

Contents

Introduction
THE CHALLENGE
DIETING THE KETO WAY

CHAPTER 1
WHAT IS A KETOGENIC DIET? 7
TYPES OF KETOGENIC DIETS
BENEFITS OF THE KETOGENIC DIET

CHAPTER 2
OVERVIEW OF THE KETOSIS PATHWAY 17
INSULIN AND KETOSIS
KETOSIS VERSUS KETOACIDOSIS

CHAPTER 3
KETO-ADAPTATION 23
DEALING WITH KETO FLU

CHAPTER 4
ARE YOU IN KETOSIS? 31
DIAGNOSTIC TESTING

CHAPTER 5
THE KETO PLAN 37
GUIDE TO HEALTHY FATS AND OILS
PLAYING IT SAFE WITH PROTEINS
KETO AND MINERALS
KETO SNACKS
FIBER
WHERE CARBS ARE HIDDEN
ADDING SUPPLEMENTS TO YOUR KETO MEAL PLAN

CHAPTER 6

GETTING STARTED 51
FOODS TO ENJOY

CHAPTER 7

INTERMITTENT FASTING 69
BENEFITS OF INTERMITTENT FASTING
KETO AND INTERMITTENT FASTING

CHAPTER 8

Vegetarians On Keto 75
WHAT IS THE VEGAN KETO DIET?
THE SOLUTION
LIMITING CARBS
IDENTIFYING HEALTHY PLANT-BASED PROTEINS
GETTING ENOUGH FAT
USING SUPPLEMENTS ON THE VEGAN KETO DIET

CHAPTER 9

YOUR GAME PLAN 87
ESTABLISHING YOUR GOALS
KETO AND EXERCISE
EATING OUT ON THE KETOGENIC DIET

CHAPTER 10

TROUBLE SHOOTING GUIDE 99

Conclusion

References

> "Eat less and move more; you will lose weight soon."

Introduction

Have you heard the slogan, "Eat less and move more; you will lose weight soon"? You have probably heard it a million times. It's everywhere you look. Some say it is the lack of willpower that stops one from shedding weight. It has become a well-known mantra that no one even bothers to question. It seems accepted without reason.

But then, *does that advice work?*

In truth, this advice is as unhelpful as a million outdated ideas we have seen before.

Looking at our lives, we are probably doing a lot of "moving" already but aren't seeing any results. Our schedules are hectic; we have kids to care for; we have a job that demands our time and even disrupts our beautiful sleep sometimes. Even with these tasks, we keep packing weight in the middle. We have our health problems in the mix, and nothing seems to help us lose all that weight.

No one intentionally wants to add weight. Excessive weight is due to several factors, like junk food, aggressive marketing, genetics, etc., and society isn't helping us with the best approach to shed weight.

Telling someone with a little more fat to eat less and move more is the same as asking an alcoholic to drink less. What we need is something entirely different. Even those crash diets don't work at all. They only help you lose a few pounds, but once you ease up on the regimen or go back to your regular meals, the weight will creep back in. Counting calories as a weight loss strategy might work, although it's not thoroughly effective. You need an all-encompassing approach because there are too many temptations along the way.

You might wonder, "How about eating what I want and exercising?" Exercise has lots of health benefits, as well as the wonders it does for our mood and brain. However, it should never be the main component of your weight loss regimen. You can eat less, move more, and exercise twice a day without losing so much. This kind of plan is hard to follow over time, which probably means that the weight will creep in soon.

THE CHALLENGE

We have the general belief that we gain weight from inactivity, poor self-control, and a bunch of other negative things. Have you tried finding out why being overweight makes one eat excessively, rather than eat less since the body is supposed to have everything it needs?

The answer lies in our body's natural feedback system. According to a doctor back in 1840, a lot of people often have damage in some regions of the brain. Since those discoveries, we have also discovered that the brain is the actual controller of how much fat is stored on a long-term basis.

So, when we have a set fat mass, the body will always look for ways to maintain that body fat composition by influencing your appetite, metabolic rate, and body heat production. Your body will also try to keep that body weight by restricting the amount of energy you lose. So, trying to alter that structured pathway through "eating less and moving more" doesn't work. The brain will act toward bringing that fat mass back up by increasing your hunger level and decreasing the amount of energy lost.

Some might be quick to point out a salient question. "Why doesn't the body try to get rid of fat mass in those of us who are overweight by increasing our metabolic rate and heat production, decreasing hunger, and helping us use stored fat as energy?" In simple terms, some enzymes regulate this. Also, signaling hormones (e.g., leptin), which travel between fat cells and the brain, are working differently. They are supposed to help the brain measure and regulate the amount of body fat we carry. In this case, those hormones are so low that you will keep filling up, and your body will keep trying to conserve energy.

Weight loss is tricky, but it can be easy if you have the right weight loss plan. Your entire weight loss plan should be focused on a diet that causes you to lose calories when you aren't out running or exercising.

The key to getting your body to work differently is by adopting procedures that control how your brain regulates fat storage. Your ideal weight loss plan must be efficient enough that you can go on for six months without having any problems. The ketogenic diet is the perfect solution.

DIETING THE KETO WAY

The ketogenic diet plan is an incredible diet you can enjoy with your entire family. Initially, it was made for kids with epilepsy many years ago. The keto diet has proven effective for both adults and kids.

If you begin the ketogenic lifestyle, your body will naturally shed weight without a fuss. Once you attain the ideal weight, you can continue maintaining that weight either with the ketogenic diet indefinitely or step back into a well-balanced meal plan. The ketogenic diet truly rocks, and I'm going to show you how to use it.

This book contains every piece of information you need about the ketogenic diet, including many strategic ways you can implement this diet on your terms. You don't have to reinvent your pantry. You only have to stick with the ingredients, strategies, tips, and hacks I'm going to show you. If you are a vegetarian, I also have lots of information for you. Within this guide, you will find everything about the vegan keto or the standard ketogenic diet plan. You can get rid of all that weight without running miles every day or stressing yourself at the gym. I believe you can become that person you've always dreamed of in only a few months.

Ready to get started? You are already on the right path!

Happy reading.

CHAPTER 1

WHAT IS A KETOGENIC DIET?

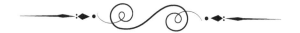

The ketogenic diet stands for a low-carb diet. It focuses on fats and not protein. So, you will cut back on carbs like white bread, pasta, and soda.

Contrary to what we know today, the ketogenic diet was initially created to help treat refractory epilepsy in kids who are difficult to control. The keto diet works by making the body burn and produce fuel from fats rather than carbohydrates.

Naturally, the body uses carbohydrates in food to make glucose, which is transported around the body, including the brain and ketone bodies.

However, when we use the ketogenic diet, we will consume less than 50 grams of carbs, which means that the body will not have enough carbohydrates for glucose conversion. Instead of eating more carbohydrates, you will eat lots of fats, which will transform your body's metabolic rate.

Again, you might be thinking, "Why fats? I thought fats are bad."

For many years, fat has been getting a lot of bad publicity from the press. But it isn't true that fats are bad. It's merely about your fat sources. According to hundreds of studies with over 900,000 participants, the entire fat category isn't to blame for all the abrogating effects linked to them. In truth, eating monounsaturated fats and saturated fats are not linked to heart disease risks.

Fats serve as one of the best forms of energy, and this is what the ketogenic diet promotes. Eating fats is very good for you. And even more, the keto diet helps in eating fresh whole foods like veggies, fish, meat, and healthy fats and oils as you get rid of processed food sources that aren't good for you.

When you want to lose weight and reap amazing benefits, the keto diet is perfect. However, you can use this diet for many other reasons. It works wonders for kids with epileptic issues. But that's not the only class of people who can use it. The ketogenic diet can also help people with acne, specific heart problems, or people with heart disease. However, it's essential you check with your doctor before using the diet.

TYPES OF KETOGENIC DIETS

All ketogenic diets concentrate on fats to bring about ketosis. Also, all the diets in this list share a lot of similarities but are different in their components.

Bear in mind that these diets are not rigid. You can figure out what works for you. Don't hesitate to ask for guidance from dietitians depending on your needs and lifestyle.

Standard Ketogenic Diet (SKD)

This diet includes very low carb, high fat, and moderate protein. In most cases, you may share your food structure in this manner: 5–10% percent carbs, 75% fat, and 20% protein. In terms of grams per day, your diet should include 40–60 g of protein and 20–50 g of carbohydrate. However, there's no limit for fat. Remember that the ketogenic diet must have a substantial array of vegetables.

Targeted Ketogenic Diet (TKD)

In TKD, you have more specific needs than weight loss. This diet is used by active individuals and athletes. It involves adding an extra 20–30 grams of carbs before and immediately after workouts to allow for enhanced recovery and higher intensity exercise.

You can eat up to 70 or 80 grams of fat with this diet. But the best option for those extra calories is grain-based foods, dairy, fruits, or sports nutrition products. This is because those extra carbs will be quickly burned off and not stored in the body.

Bear in mind that those extra carbs might decrease if you aren't doing high-intensity exercise. So, in a targeted keto diet, you can have 20% protein, 10–15% carbs, and 65–70% fat.

Cyclical Ketogenic Diet (CKD)

CKD involves cycling in and out of ketosis. For instance, you can have two non-keto days and five days of traditional diet every week.

This diet helps you enjoy a more balanced diet on non-keto days and can help people who save up to go crazy, especially on weekends to have more fun. To gain the right results, stick with whole, carb-rich foods on your off days.

High-Protein Ketogenic Diet (HPKD)

HPKD further restricts carb content but includes eating more protein to about 120 grams of protein and 130 grams of fat per day. In this case, carbs will be less than 10% daily. Some people like using this diet because it seems easier to follow. However, this diet might not result in ketosis since the proteins work exactly like carbs and will be converted to glucose for fuel. Weight loss can occur, but people at risk of kidney and liver-related problems shouldn't use this variant.

MCT Ketogenic Diet

In this case, you might follow the standard ketogenic diet, but you will focus on getting medium-chain triglycerides (MCTs), which will boost the fat content in your diet. You can find MCTs in coconut oil, MCT emulsion liquids, and MCT oil. When used appropriately, this diet can help epileptic conditions and allow people to consume more carbohydrates and protein while going into ketosis. Be aware that MCTs can cause diarrhea or stomach upset if consumed in large quantities. To prevent this, make sure your meals have equal portions of non-MCT fat and MCTs.

BENEFITS OF THE KETOGENIC DIET

There are so many amazing benefits of the ketogenic diet. Most of these benefits are backed by research, while some still have some controversies.

1. Weight loss

The keto diet is so satisfying even as it helps you lose weight, and it doesn't require counting calories. According to a study, the ketogenic diet resulted in 2.2 times more weight loss for people when compared with another calorie-restricted, low-fat diet.

The ketogenic diet improves your triglyceride and HDL cholesterol levels. In addition to helping you lose weight efficiently, it lowers your blood sugar levels and improves your insulin sensitivity, which plays a crucial role in weight loss. In fact, you can lose more weight within the first three to six months of keto, therefore, gaining a very stable and balanced weight.

2. Excellent for prediabetes and diabetes

Diabetes causes impaired insulin function, high blood sugar, and changes in body metabolism. The ketogenic diet is known for improving all of these conditions. It also helps one to lose excess fat linked to a diabetic ailment and helps improve insulin sensitivity by over 75%. But that's not all; the ketogenic diet can even reverse type 2 diabetes and prediabetes.

3. Neurological conditions

The ketogenic diet is an established and powerful tool for treating neurological diseases like epilepsy. It can cause considerable reductions in seizures in children with epilepsy. Also, it helps metabolic function and can improve heart conditions, including heart disease, high blood pressure, and kidney disease.

4. Cancer

The ketogenic diet has gotten a reputation in treating several cancer conditions and reducing tumor growth. It can be used as an antitumor chemotherapy treatment or a supportive cancer treatment.

5. Alzheimer's disease

The keto diet can minimize Alzheimer's disease and even slow its progression. The keto diet can help you focus better and improves memory. This is because there is a higher intake of healthy fats with omega-3, which is necessary for enhancing mood and learning ability.

6. Brain injuries and epilepsy

According to some research, the keto diet is beneficial for the treatment of concussions and can help recovery after a brain injury. The brain functions more efficiently when ketones are used as fuel rather than sugar, and these ketones also have inhibitory effects on the nerve cells, making it possible for the person to have fewer seizures, less autism-like behavior, and enhanced brain function.

7. Acne

The ketogenic diet can help eradicate acne because it lowers insulin levels and helps cultivate habits of eating less processed foods or sugar. Also, the keto diet improves your appetite by making you feel full for a long time, reducing cravings, and eradicating sugary food preferences.

8. Polycystic ovary syndrome

Because the keto diet can help improve insulin levels, it can play a fantastic role in treating polycystic ovary syndrome. The diet is also efficient in treating yeast infections and thrush, which are usually associated with lower blood sugar.

9. Parkinson's disease

Studies have equally shown that the keto diet can improve symptoms associated with Parkinson's disease.

10. Exercise

You can also exercise on keto. However, the ketogenic

diet helps endurance athletes, i.e., cyclists, runners, and many more. It can improve their muscle-fat ratio over time and raise the amount of oxygen retained by the body when working hard.

Why Keto Stands Out Among Other Popular Diet Plans

Big plans like Paleo and Atkins are efficient, but the keto diet stands out for many reasons. It is super-effective in restricting carbs without calculating calories, which is twice as much as we can see with the Paleo or Atkins diet.

It is the only diet among all three that causes ketosis and includes more fats and oils than the other diets. Keto also brings in the powers of the dairy. However, the keto diet, unlike those other diets, restricts the consumption of fruits, grains, beans, and legumes. It's equally a straightforward diet to follow over a long time without causing unnecessary harm to your body.

Besides, keto is safe for most people. But if you breastfeed or are taking medications for diabetes or high blood pressure, your doctor will want to watch you or give you medicines while on the keto diet. That's because there are controversies over the medications that will work for you with those conditions when you are on the keto diet. However, it's still safe for you. All you have to do is let your doctor know your plans.

CHAPTER 2
OVERVIEW OF THE KETOSIS PATHWAY

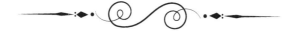

Why does the ketogenic diet work incredibly well in areas where other diets don't work? How does it enable our body to use up our fat stores rather than convert the food we are giving it to glucose?

The reason is the ketosis pathway.

When you eat food, it provides the fuel that your body uses for everyday activities both internally and externally, as well as helps the body grow. However, your body can run on three primary fuels: fats, proteins, and carbohydrates. Generally, the main source of this fuel is carbohydrates. All of these nutrients will undergo the same kind of chemical reaction, with oxygen as a component to bring about energy and some waste products. When all three of these fuels are metabolized for energy, carbohydrates are used first because they are available and more comfortable to metabolize, followed by fats and lastly, protein. Typically, carbs will be used or depleted a few hours after eating, and this is why we frequently eat on that kind of diet.

However, owing to the metabolism of carbohydrates, the body will continue to store excess calories it doesn't need to have energy later in two ways: glycogenesis and lipogenesis.

Glycogenesis is the process of converting and storing excess glucose in the liver and muscles as glycogen, while **lipogenesis** is the conversion of that stored glycogen into fats. In the end, the body can store fats that may give us the ability to sustain ourselves for weeks to months without adequate food. In our typical western diet, the body will continue storing excess glucose through those pathways for future use.

By contrast, when we restrict our carbohydrate intake and raise the proportion of fats, the body will be forced to metabolize the fats into highly efficient molecules called ketones. These ketones are synthesized after the breakdown of fats into fatty acid and glycerol, which can be used directly as fuel in many cells throughout the body but not used as energy by the brain. To meet the needs of the brain, the fatty acid and glycerol will enter the liver, where they can be converted to sugar and ketones. In more specific terms, the glycerol goes through the process of gluconeogenesis, while the fatty acids go through the process of **ketogenesis** as it converts to ketone bodies.

As a result of ketogenesis, the body produces a ketone component called acetoacetate that is broken into two types of ketone bodies: beta-hydroxybutyrate (BHB), which is a more efficient fuel source, and acetone, which will be excreted as waste and is responsible for the fruity breath ketogenic dieters have. Over time, the body will continue expelling ketone bodies as acetone, which can be measured to track your ketone levels. However, the body will also create glucose, because ketones alone cannot meet the energy needs of the brain and body. In this case, the liver uses a different pathway called **gluconeogenesis.** The amino acids, glycerol, and lactate will be converted into sugar to meet the glucose needs of the body.

The **ketogenesis** and **gluconeogenesis** pathways will work together as you continue to restrict carbohydrates, but this does not mean your ketone levels will steadily increase. If you overeat protein, it will get in the way of ketosis and enhance the needs of gluconeogenesis and the production of more sugar. That is why it is vital to regulate your protein intake when on the keto diet.

Therefore, the ketogenic diet mimics the starvation or fasting state by denying the body essential carbohydrates for fuel, forcing it to metabolize fats. As you continue using the ketogenic diet, here's what happens to you:

- You will lose more body fat and weight without fear of gaining it back.
- You will have better cholesterol levels.
- Your blood sugar will reduce.
- Your appetite for the wrong foods will decrease.
- Your triglyceride levels will reduce.
- There will be significant blood pressure reductions.

INSULIN AND KETOSIS

Insulin hormone is responsible for a lot of things, particularly the metabolism of sugar. So, it suppresses the production of ketones. The consumption of sugar activates the creation of this hormone. However, it can be involved in a bit of a problem, particularly for people with type 2 diabetes.

Our body produces insulin for the adequate metabolism of sugar from the blood into energy used by cells and brain. In this case, we are sensitive to the metabolic signals brought by insulin (insulin sensitivity). When we become insulin resistant, the cells will reject the actions of insulin (insulin resistant), leading to an accumulation of sugar in the bloodstream, which is dangerous and diagnosed as type 2 diabetes.

So, when we minimize our sugar intake, we are reducing the production of insulin in the body. However, we should also watch our protein intake because too much protein can also trigger an insulin spike. With the generation of ketones other than the production of insulin, the blood sugar will reduce, and those insulin resistant problems can be efficiently regulated. This is the reason why the ketogenic diet can be effectively used to reverse the issues of prediabetes and type 2 diabetes.

However, with medications alongside, the ketogenic diet must be effectively monitored, as this diet can reduce insulin levels to the point where you risk developing low blood sugar, which is diagnosed as hypoglycemia.

KETOSIS VERSUS KETOACIDOSIS

In ketosis and ketoacidosis, ketones are produced in the body. However, ketoacidosis is a lethal process that can be life-threatening. Ketosis occurs when the body begins burning fat instead of glucose, which is the aim of the ketogenic diet. Ketoacidosis occurs when the body produces dangerously high ketones. This can happen when there is type 2 and type 1 diabetes, especially when there is no control of the blood sugar levels. This is one of the reasons you need to track your ketone levels as you progress with the diet. Look out for symptoms such as:

- Dry or flushed skin
- Exhaustion
- High blood glucose levels
- High levels of ketones in the urine
- Stomach pain
- Trouble breathing
- Nausea and vomiting
- Loss of consciousness
- Confusion and difficulty in paying attention

The best way to be sure whether you are in ketosis or ketoacidosis is by checking your blood ketone levels. If you have diabetes, then you should take your testing seriously and report to your doctor when you see any abnormalities.

CHAPTER 3
KETO-ADAPTATION

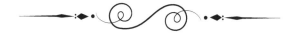

Keto-adaptation, sometimes called fat-adaptation, is the process your body goes through when you use the keto diet to convert its primary source of fuel from glucose to fat. This occurs when the stores of glycogen are depleted and the body has begun adapting to the use of fats and ketones. This transition occurs within two to seven days of commencing the diet. In some people, it can take up to three weeks, after which you begin to see the positive aspects of keto-adaptation.

Some factors can also slow down your adaptation process. Your age, daily fat and protein intake, carb intake, exercise, and metabolism are some of those factors. That's because your body must first use up its glycogen stores before it begins entering the ketogenic pathway. If you overindulge in carbs or proteins, you will slow down the adaptation process. However, some people can enter ketosis while eating up to 90 grams of carbs a day, even if the ideal weight of carbs for the keto diet is 50 grams. Some people even need fewer carbs (as low as 25 grams) per day to enter ketosis. If you are struggling with keto-adaptation, then you should try reducing your carb intake below 50 grams.

Also, if you overeat protein or eat too little fat, it might slow down the process. Therefore, it's essential to balance your diet as instructed in later chapters. You should also watch your exercise, sleep, and stress rate. If you want to enter ketosis faster, then you should consider adding some exercise to the mix, as this helps your body empty carbs more quickly. You can also influence the keto pathway by sticking to a fasting schedule. This can also help hasten your keto-adaptation process.

Here are some more tips to help you enter ketosis faster.

- Try preparing your meals rather than eating out.

- Eat between 20 to 50 grams of carbs per day.
- Check for hidden carbs, especially in condiments, dressing, and sauces.
- Try using *intermittent fasting*.
- Add physical activity to the mix.
- Use a medium-chain triglyceride (MCT) supplement.
- Track your ketone levels.

Signs of Keto-Adaptation

You might be able to get into ketosis during the first few days or weeks, but this does not mean you are now entirely keto-adapted. You can figure out when you are in ketosis using the signs and symptoms in the next chapter, but you need a more subjective measurement to figure out your adaptation levels. Here are various ways you can use in checking.

1. Higher energy levels

Glucose energy levels get depleted quickly. This is why we usually have sugar crashes or sugar highs on those kinds of diets. When you have adapted to a fat-burning diet, you won't have swings in energy levels. You will have plenty of body fat to burn at all times, and even when you skip meals, there won't be problems.

2. Reduced cravings

You will crave a lot of things for the first few weeks. This is because sugar is physically addictive, and cutting it out of your diet might make you miserable for some days (keto flu). But once you are fat-adapted, your hunger levels will be suppressed, and you won't crave sugary snacks.

3. A clear mind

During the first few weeks, you might also experience a temporary dip in brain and energy functions. This means you might have brain fog and a few headaches, but once you are fat-adapted, these effects will subside, and you will have enhanced focus.

4. Higher endurance levels

Due to sugar highs and crashes, a lot of people on the glucose diet don't have long physical endurance. Fat-adaptation boosts physical endurance capacity and can be so amazing when you are using high-intensity workouts.

5. Loss of body fat

You will lose weight in the first few days, but that's only water weight from stored glycogen. When your body begins to burn fat, which usually occurs after four weeks of keto dieting, then you can finally say that you are fat-adapted.

Fat-adaptation doesn't happen overnight. You have to

deal with the keto flu stage before you become fat-adapted.

DEALING WITH KETO FLU

The keto flu is symptoms you will see once you begin withdrawing from carbs. The intensity of this process can be high if you quickly jump into the keto diet. These signs can pop up quickly in as little as two days once you begin cutting back on carbs. Some of the symptoms you have may include:

- Constipation
- Nausea and vomiting
- Diarrhea
- Headache
- Irritability
- Muscle cramps
- Stomach pain
- Difficulty sleeping
- Sugar cravings
- Weakness

These symptoms can make you miserable. But you can get rid of them using the following tips:

- Drinks lots of water
- Avoid strenuous exercise
- Eat food that is high in potassium, like avocados and

green leafy veggies
- Get enough sleep
- Reduce your intake of caffeine
- Make sure your fat sources are high enough
- Get enough salt and electrolytes

Adverse Effects to Avoid

Besides the keto flu, there are other side effects you have to look out for. These side effects may require you to adjust or even discontinue the diet. When you witness any of these symptoms, you must consult your doctor for the next line of action. Some of them include:

1. **Hyperacidosis:** This occurs when your ketone levels are too high. They result from becoming ill or being overactive. In these cases, you might only need rehydration or may have to adjust the diet.
2. **Kidney stones:** If you are not taking enough fluids, you may risk developing kidney stones. Look out for difficulty in urination, blood in the urine, or severe back pain. You may need to adjust the diet or even discontinue it.
3. **Hypercholesterolemia:** Not everyone can metabolize fat efficiently. In such cases, lipid levels may go up. Most doctors may recommend using a mineral supplement to combat this problem or adjusting your fat intake.
4. **Hypoglycemia:** This is also known as low blood

sugar. This can occur alongside increased levels of ketones and reduced levels of insulin. It's a condition you must look out for, especially when diabetic. You may have to adjust your diet or even stop it when necessary.

5. **Osteoporosis:** Some people have experienced osteoporosis due to this diet. You can avoid it by taking a vitamin and calcium supplement.

6. **Pancreatitis:** The pancreas is primarily responsible for breaking down fat. If your pancreas cannot handle the increased fat intake, it may become swollen or inflamed, and the entire gastrointestinal system will stop working. In this case, you may experience severe abdominal discomfort, and your abdomen might be too tender to touch. If you experience it, you must stop the diet immediately and never attempt it again.

CHAPTER 4
ARE YOU IN KETOSIS?

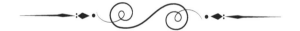

Unlike many other diet plans, the keto diet has legitimate signals to tell you when it's working. This means when your liver begins to produce a high number of ketones to supply energy to your brain, you will see particular symptoms. However, for some people, it might be difficult detecting these symptoms. In those cases, it's better to test for it. Nevertheless, here are some signs you might have:

Bad Breath

Although this is technically a fruity smell, some might call it bad breath. What causes your breathing to take on that fruity smell is the elevated ketone levels, which will find ways to exit your body through your urine and breath. Many people on the keto diet might choose to wash their mouth several times during the day to avoid this, as it can be less than ideal for their social lives. You can also use gum, but be sure that it is sugar-free and low carb, otherwise it may reduce your ketone levels and enhance your blood sugar levels. Even when you don't have noticeable fruity breath, it is possible to test your ketone levels using breath analyzers.

Suppressed Appetite

When your body has successfully adapted to the ketogenic diet, you might begin experiencing reduced cravings for food. This is particularly higher when you are in ketosis because the ketones might be sending signals to your brain to reduce your appetite. So, when you feel full and don't need to eat as often as you felt at the beginning of the diet plan, then you might be in ketosis.

Heightened Focus and Energy

After you have stopped experiencing the keto flu, you

may begin to experience increased energy and focus. That's because your body has adapted to burning more fat as fuel rather than carbs. So, since your brain is probably burning ketones rather than glucose, you might begin to focus more on other activities. Also, your energy levels will be more stable throughout the day.

Digestive Problems

Switching out of your regular meal plan to the keto diet requires time for your digestive system to switch as well. So, you may have constipation or diarrhea during the early stages. To combat these issues, ensure that you are eating lots of low-carb veggies with plenty of fiber. Also, ensure that your diet is as diverse as possible. Don't eat a few meal recipes throughout the week, or you might become deficient in some essential nutrients.

Insomnia

You might also have trouble sleeping for the first few weeks. That's your brain trying to swap away from its normal glucose "meal." However, when you adapt to the diet, you will begin to sleep better.

Weight Loss

This is one of the visible signs you will see. As soon as you enter ketosis, your body will begin losing weight rapidly. You can see this weight loss in as little as the first week. There is belief that the rapid weight loss you see in the first week is fat loss. But it isn't because you will only lose water and stored carbs. After the first week, your body will begin losing weight consistently, as long as you continue your diet.

Enhanced Ketones in Urine and Blood

You will also reduce blood sugar levels and have increased ketone levels. You can't see this except through the use of a specialized meter that tests your blood ketone levels. You can also measure ketone levels by testing samples of your urine.

DIAGNOSTIC TESTING

Besides the prominent symptoms, you can still measure your ketone levels to be very sure that you are in ketosis. This is more accurate than merely checking for those signs. However, tests require a little spending on your part. You can begin testing your ketone levels after the first two or three days, but it's ideal to wait for up to a week. That's because ketosis might take about two to seven days, but some people don't start until after two weeks. At the point you enter ketosis, you might be done with the keto flu and the adaptation process. Before you begin measuring, you can look out for the symptoms mentioned earlier as guidance. That way, you won't waste a few dollars on the first few kits. You can monitor the number of ketones in your body in several ways, including:

1. **Ketone monitor:** This is far more accurate than any other method. It requires a little blood to test your blood ketone levels. Many of these ketone monitors work like blood sugar monitors and require a tiny pinprick of blood from your finger onto a test strip. The ketone meter tests for beta-hydroxybutyrate in your blood. There are many blood meters that you can buy. However, the strips are a little expensive and can add up if you decide to test multiple times a day, which isn't relevant. When testing, you should look for ketone levels above 0.3 mmol/L, although some experts consider having higher levels between 0.5 and 3.0 mmol/l optimal.

2. **Urine testing strips:** These are commonly used, more comfortable, and cheaper than the ketone monitor. When you use these strips, they will change colors to indicate the acetoacetate in your urine. But these strips are not accurate all the time. That's because you might be dehydrated or even overhydrated. Also, as your body begins to adapt to the process, your urine levels may not reflect the ketones in your body.

3. **Breath testing strips:** Breath testing strips are more affordable than any other option because you

won't have to replace strips. They only test for lower ketone levels and are not accurate for higher ketone levels. So, you can think about switching from breath testing strips after the first few weeks, as they might not be instrumental after that.

Look out for ketone levels above 3.0 mmol/L. If you see such levels of ketones, then you need to consult your doctor because such levels are dangerous, especially if you have diabetes and you are on insulin.

CHAPTER 5
THE KETO PLAN

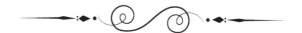

Your standard diet usually involves 35% fat, 15% protein, and 50% carbs. In contrast, the keto diet includes 70% high-quality fat, 20% protein, and 10% carbs. Therefore, your goal isn't to extremely increase your protein levels, but to enhance your fat levels. Some people may not consider counting calories on the keto diet. It's not compulsory, as long as you are effectively watching your intake. But you must try not to cheat yourself out of ketosis by bringing in more carbs. The only way to increase calories should be by increasing your fat intake, and you should reduce calories by decreasing your protein and carbohydrate intake.

When beginning your keto diet, make sure you clean out your pantry of those starchy temptations. Plan your meals so you won't have to cook the same food more than once. You need to make sure you are getting your calories from the right places. Bear in mind that all calories aren't equal. Your 20% protein-calories should come from omega-rich sources. Your fat sources should be equally healthy, while your carbs must be healthy as well. In this section, we will distinguish unhealthy food sources from healthy ones so that you can plan your keto diet efficiently.

GUIDE TO HEALTHY FATS AND OILS

Fats add richness to your food and can help you feel satisfied quickly. Fat also regulates immunity and inflammation alongside providing access to fat-soluble vitamins, like vitamins A, D, E, and K. Fats are essential for your skin, hair, and most of your body cells.

In the keto diet, you need saturated fats, monounsaturated fats, and polyunsaturated fats, but your polyunsaturated fats should be strictly from unprocessed food stores.

Processed polyunsaturated fats are those found in margarine and vegetable oils. Your polyunsaturated fat sources should be fatty fish, pastured eggs, grass-fed meats, algae, chia seeds, flaxseeds, walnuts, and hemp seeds.

For monounsaturated fats, you can get them from nuts, avocados/avocado oil, lard, tallow, and olive oil, while saturated fats can come from cream, ghee, coconut oil, lard, tallow, and butter.

Nevertheless, no food contains 100% saturated, monounsaturated, and polyunsaturated fats. In truth, some foods contain predominantly one type of fat. So, it's crucial you mix in a little of everything. Avoid processed seed and vegetable oils, such as canola, corn, soybean oil, sunflower, and safflower oils. They can be harmful to you. However, you shouldn't overdo your fat content. If you eat too many fats, it might stop weight loss or even slow down your metabolic rates. Eat enough fats, but don't make a mistake of eating too little carbs and fat at the same time. If you are having trouble figuring out how to add fat to your diet, use these strategies:

- Use whole full-fat sources, like eggs and avocados.
- Cook with fats.
- Use different fats to achieve a variety of flavors.
- Top meals with dressing, sauces, oil, or butter.
- Top meals with high-fat foods, like avocados.
- Do your best to avoid snacks, but if you must eat

them, make sure it's either nuts, cheese, hard-boiled eggs, or other real fat foods.
- You can also add fat to your tea or coffee.

PLAYING IT SAFE WITH PROTEINS

Proteins are made of smaller components known as amino acids. Our body can produce about twenty amino acids, but nine of them can only be consumed from food. Protein is vital in your keto diet because it helps with muscle repair and growth.

You also need proteins for sustaining the health of your nails, bones, hair, skin, and internal organs. It is also essential for creating enzymes and hormones. In keto, you have to make sure you aren't having too much protein or too little protein. It should be moderate. Ideally, you should have between 1.2 to 1.7 grams per kg of body weight of protein daily. If you are an athlete, you may need up to 2.0 grams of proteins per kg of body weight. Some people who are underweight or recovering from surgery, injury, or illness may need up to 2.0 grams per kg of body weight.

Nevertheless, you should aim for 20 to 30 grams of protein at each meal to make sure you have all the amino acids you need. It's often better to spread out your protein intake with meals than consuming all of it at once. If you are over sixty-five, then you need a minimum of 1.2 kg per body weight of protein to decrease the loss of strength, weakness, or frailty.

If you are an intermittent faster, you may consider increasing protein portions at the two meals you are eating to meet the mark. You can also get proteins from nuts and seeds, but bear in mind that although they look small, their contents can add up quickly. If you are not getting enough protein, here are some of the signs you may see:

- Feeling tired and weak all the time
- Having brain fog despite using MCT oils
- Having peeling skin, brittle nails, or thinning hair
- Constant craving of sweets after the first week
- Unable to lose weight or gaining weight
- Feeling sick all the time
- Having swollen ankles, feet, or legs
- Losing muscle mass

Make sure you are getting enough protein, but don't overdo it. Luckily, if you focus on eating whole-based foods with enough fat and non-starchy vegetables, you won't go overboard with protein.

KETO AND MINERALS

There are five most essential minerals you need on

your keto diet. These include sodium, potassium, magnesium, phosphorus, and calcium. You also need trace minerals in a smaller amount, such as zinc, selenium, molybdenum, manganese, iron, copper, cobalt, and iodine. Usually, you won't have deficiencies in copper, zinc, manganese, molybdenum, or phosphorus since you can get those from seeds, seafood, nuts, and green veggies. However, minerals like calcium, potassium, magnesium, and iron are difficult to achieve at optimal levels. In most cases, you may need supplementation, as discussed in the next chapter.

When you begin keto, you will need more calcium and potassium to help with the keto-adaptation phase. It's advised that you get up to 1,000 mg of calcium and 5,000 mg of potassium per day from your food or by using a supplement. Oily fish, broccoli, turnip greens, kale, and almond milk are some excellent ways to replenish your calcium and potassium stores. But supplementation is necessary. For iodine, you can get all you need from seaweeds or by eating dairy, eggs, and white fish. Iron is contained in oysters, eggs, liver, and red meat. Nuts, seeds, and edible darker greens, like chard and spinach, can replenish your magnesium stores. You can also get about 10% of your daily magnesium requirements by using yogurt and avocado. You may need a bit of selenium, which you can find in brazil nuts; a single one is enough for your daily selenium needs.

In recent years, sodium has been getting a bad reputation, particularly with its links to heart health. You don't need high sodium levels, as it can raise your blood pressure. But those kinds of levels can only be achieved from eating highly processed foods. If you follow the keto diet strategically by using fresh, whole foods, you may not have too little or too low sodium levels. The first week of keto will be marked by a high loss in water and sodium. You can top your sodium levels by using 1 to 2 tablespoons of quality salt per day and lots of water. You can also use salted, smoked, or cured meat, fish, and bacon to meet your sodium needs. Beware of cheap table salt because it contains maltodextrin, which is a sugar used in stabilizing it.

KETO SNACKS

You can sometimes snack on the keto diet, but it's essential that it doesn't happen every day. For the best part, the keto food recipes can keep hunger at bay, hours after meals. If, for any reason, you wish to snack, then you should make sure that there are more fats in your snacks.

Some people make the mistake of having too many keto cookies or keto brownies for snacks. They should be used only on great occasions and not as a staple in your diet. Also, never snack on vitamin water, fruit juice, cashew nuts, cafe lattes, grapes, or bananas. The most horrible choices you shouldn't make are snacking on nachos, chips, or chocolate bars. They are awful for your health and will pull you out of ketosis. The good news is that the keto diet will reduce those cravings, so you won't even miss them.

Try as much as possible not to snack so much. Indulging in it will add excess calories into your diet, which may become converted to a more natural fuel source for the body. If you must snack, then use these options:

1. **Whole foods**

You can snack on nuts, like brazil nuts, pecan nuts, and macadamia nuts. You can also snack on boiled eggs, cold cuts, olives, and avocadoes. They are the best and tasty options for keeping hunger at bay and filling yourself with healthy fats.

2. **Veggie sticks**

You can snack on veggie sticks made from the lowest carb vegetables, like cucumber, celery low-carb dip sauce, or peppers (green, yellow, and red pepper). You can also snack on eggplants, tomato, or asparagus. However, avoid snacking on carrots, as they have higher carbs and might put you above your daily limits. Never snack on potato chips, parsnip, and other root food products.

3. Berries and cream

You can snack on berries and cream occasionally. But make sure you are only using modest amounts of frozen or fresh berries because too many of them can knock you out of ketosis. Generally, raspberries, blackberries, and strawberries are okay, but blueberries are a lot higher in carbs.

4. Chocolates

Give yourself a chocolate treat occasionally as long as your choice has over 70% or 85% cacao. The former has only 3.5g carbs per square, while the latter has 2 grams per square. Don't snack on white chocolate, milk chocolate, or dark chocolate.

5. Other snacks

You can also snack on pork rinds, biltong, or beef jerky. Choose those with the lowest carbs. You can also snack on pili nuts, parmesan chips, or coconut oil.

FIBER

Fiber is needed for your gut health and long-term nutrition. This can be difficult because most high-fiber foods are also high in carbs. Here are some strategies you can use to gain enough fiber without preventing or slowing ketosis:

- Eat a lot of leafy veggies.
- Use mineral or multivitamin supplements.
- Eat foods with lots of minerals and electrolytes.
- Make sure you drink a lot of water.
- Use low-carb, "keto-friendly" packaged foods.
- Have more salads in your diet.
- Add roasted or sautéed vegetables.
- Dress your food with dips and dressings made from leafy greens.

WHERE CARBS ARE HIDDEN

If you are struggling with ketosis, it might be because you have more carbs without knowing it. A lot of common foods contain more carbs than we imagine. So, it's important you watch out for them. Some food sources with hidden carbs include:

1. **Yogurt:** Aim for whole milk or full-fat Greek yogurt rather than their low-fat, fruit-flavored counterparts.
2. **Salad dressing:** If you aren't sure of the amount of sugar in your salad dressing, then you should use vinegar or olive oil.
3. **Chestnuts:** Chestnuts can have up to 15g of carbs per serving.
4. **Low-fat or fat-free:** Avoid food products with these labels. They might be low in fat, but they usually have more carbs.

5. **Ketchup and tomato sauce:** There are carbs and hidden sugars in tomato products.
6. **Milk substitutes:** Be careful of soy or almond milk, as they might have hidden carbs.
7. **No added sugar or sugar-free:** Food products with these labels, such as raisins or fruit juice, have high sugar content.
8. **Sweeteners:** Be careful when using molasses, honey, nectar, agave, and high fructose corn syrup.
9. **Seasoning and sauces:** Make sure you know the number of carbs in your sauces and seasoning. Be careful of blended spices.
10. **Supplements and protein bars:** Avoid flavored, chewable, or coated supplements and protein bars because they contain a high level of carbs.
11. **Meats and eggs:** Be sure of the carbs in your eggs and meats. Keto-friendly meats are goat, lamb, pork cuts, poultry, and beef.

ADDING SUPPLEMENTS TO YOUR KETO MEAL PLAN

When faced with the question of whether you should add supplements to your keto meal plan or stick to the basics, the short answer is that supplements can help make your diet a lot easier.

The ketogenic diet is so unique that it will transform

your default energy source away from carbs by using a low-carb diet. And when that switch happens, your gallbladder and liver will release all the stored fats in your body, creating an alternative source of energy. Supplements can hasten the pathway to prevent any hitch. They can help by making up for the lack of vitamins and minerals you meet when you have the keto flu. Besides, the keto diet doesn't allow all kinds of fruits and starchy vegetables, so your mineral and vitamin stores might not be enough. Ultimately, supplements will make up for the lack of nutrients in your keto diet and support your weight loss efforts. There are many kinds of supplements you can use, except if you are using the vegan keto meal plan; you can use these keto supplements listed below:

1. **Electrolytes**

Adding salts and other minerals to your diet is essential, especially when starting on the keto diet. This is because your diet might be missing out on some critical minerals, which may result in the keto flu. To avoid or minimize the effects of the keto flu, as well as control your nerve and muscle function, you need electrolytes. You can take sodium, magnesium, potassium, and calcium supplements. A rule of thumb is to have 2,300 mg of sodium, 320 mg of magnesium, and 1,000 mg of calcium.

2. **Vitamin D**

Vitamin D is both a hormone and nutrient in your body. A lot of food products have it, although it's hard to get it from those sources alone. Staying in sunny areas can also boost your sources, but waiting too long in the sun puts you at risk of cancer. Since you will be on the ketogenic diet, you will have higher chances of having vitamin D deficiency. You can use fortified dairy products, but it is recommended you supplement with 400 IU per day.

3. MCT oil

MCT means medium-chain triglycerides. They are a type of fat used by the body to store energy instantly instead of storing them as fat. With MCTs, your body can produce ketones quickly, which provides a more efficient way of entering ketosis. You can get MCTs from butter, cheese, coconut oil, or yogurt. But it's better to get a more concentrated dose from MCT oil or MCT oil powder.

4. Collagen

You can also take collagen supplements to improve muscle growth and recovery. This supplement will also support your brain health, optimize your metabolic functions, and improve your overall sleep quality. It's equally excellent for enhancing the integrity and function of your tendons, ligaments, joints, and bones.

CHAPTER 6
GETTING STARTED

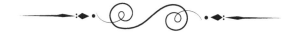

The ketogenic diet follows a high-fat, low-carb, and moderate-protein diet. By now, you must have realized that there are different kinds of carbohydrates and that not all carbohydrates are worth it for the ketogenic diet. This means that even when you try to add them in smaller amounts, you are better off using other carb sources. You need carbs that won't give you a surge of insulin, which will ruin the chances of ketosis occurring.

Also, you need quality fat, which also means that your source of fat equally matters. In this section, I will help you figure out the kind of food substances that work when following the ketogenic diet. Your content depends on the type of ketogenic diet you want to use. In this guide, we will stick to the standard ketogenic diet, and you can personalize it as you want.

FOODS TO ENJOY

Non-starchy Vegetables

In terms of the ketogenic diet, you can't eat all kinds of vegetables. You need vegetable sources that are rich in fiber, vitamins, and minerals but low in carbs. These kinds of plants are called non-starchy vegetables. Both starchy and non-starchy vegetables are rich in vitamins, minerals, fiber, and antioxidants, but their key differences are their carbohydrate content. According to U.S. health agencies, you need 2.5 cups of vegetables a day, both non-starchy and starchy types. But in the ketogenic diet, you must stick to the non-starchy kinds listed below and reduce the intake based on the number of calories you need.

For the Non-starchy Vegetable:

1 Serving size for non-starchy vegetables = 2–3 cups raw leafy greens = ½ cup cooked or 1 cup raw other non-starchy vegetables = approximately 25 calories.

- Leafy greens
- Beet
- Dandelion
- Arugula
- Collard
- Endive
- Escarole
- Kale
- Spinach
- Swiss chard
- Radicchio
- Watercress
- Asparagus
- Bamboo shoots
- Artichoke & Jerusalem artichoke
- Broccoli
- Brussels sprouts
- Celery
- Celery roots
- Eggplants
- Cucumber
- Green or String beans

- Cabbage (green, nappa, red, bok choy, savoy)
- Bean sprouts
- Hearts of palm
- Bitter melon
- Cactus
- Okra
- Onion (white, yellow, red, scallions, shallot, green, spring, brown)
- Sauerkraut
- Sea plants (kelp, nori, kombu, dulse, arame)
- Tomatoes
- Turnips
- Water chestnuts
- Leeks
- Mushrooms
- Radishes
- Pepper (Sweet, poblano, jalapeno, bell)
- Rutabaga
- Sugar snap peas and snow peas
- Summer squash (patty pan, zucchini, spaghetti, delicata, yellow, crookneck)
- Jicama
- Chayote
- Kimchi
- Kohlrabi

Dairy

You can also eat dairy products in the ketogenic diet. But when you buy them, it's necessary to keep in mind that you need those with higher fat content and not higher carb content. Look out for preservatives, additives, and all those other things that could be hiding the carbs. Make sure you aren't allergic or sensitive to the dairy products you buy. If you check out for hidden carbs thoroughly, you can even use thick yogurts, sour cream, or rich cheese in your diet. Therefore, not all forms of dairy are suitable for the keto lifestyle. It is recommended that you use full-fat dairy products as long as their carb contents are low. Here are some dairy products you can add:

1. **Milk:** There are three kinds—dry milk, evaporated milk, and milk. Dry milk and evaporated milk can't be used since they have 10% and 50% lactose respectively. Lactose still converts to glucose in the blood, so you don't need much of it. Regular milk contains 5% lactose, and 1 cup of it should be enough to provide 100 to 150 calories.

2. **Cheese:** Go for fattier, harder varieties of cheese. This includes gouda, cheddar cheese, swiss cheese, feta cheese, and parmesan. They have high amounts of fats, low carbs, and moderate quantities of calcium, vitamin A, vitamin B, and proteins.

3. **Cream:** Unlike popular notions, creams contain high fat, but you have to watch out for additives. You need partially fermented cream because it has less lactose than its unfermented counterparts.
4. **Yogurt:** Full-fat yogurts are ideal here. They are lower in fat than other dairy products, but they contain a good deal of protein and low lactose content. Yogurts also aid digestion. A ½ cup of yogurt gives 100–150 calories.
5. **Butter: Butter** is a must in the keto diet. It is lactose-free and low in protein. You are free to spread, bake, or cook with it.

Protein

Protein is important for going keto, so you have to monitor your intake so that it stays on the right side. Most ketogenic food plans will include eggs or meat in the diet. Excessive protein causes the body to break down the protein into fuel, which ultimately leads out of ketosis.

For Proteins

1 Serving = approximately 150 calories

It includes:

- Cheese:
  - Goat: 2 oz.
  - Mozzarella: 2 oz. or shredded, ½ cup

GETTING STARTED

- Ricotta: 1/3 cup
- Feta: 2 oz.
- Cottage: 3/4 cup

- Bacon: (2 slices)
- Buffalo: 3 oz.; other beef, 3 oz.
- Cornish hen: 4 oz.
- Egg whites: 1 cup
- Eggs, whole: 2
- Chicken, white or dark meat: 3 oz.
- Elk: 3 oz.
- Venison: 3 oz.
- Shellfish (crabs, lobster, clams, mussels, oysters, scallops): 4–5 oz.
- Pork, tenderloin: 2 oz.
- Liver: 3 oz.
- Lamb (chop, leg, or lean roast): 3 oz.
- Fish:

- Tuna

- Skipjack: 4 oz.
- Yellowtail: 4 oz.
- Solid light, chunk light, or canned (in oil or water): 4 oz.

- Trout: 4 oz.
- Sardines (in oil or water): 3 oz.
- Mackerel: 2 oz.

- o Herring: 3 oz.
- o Salmon

- ➢ Fresh: 3 oz.
- ➢ Smoked: 3 oz.
- ➢ Canned: 3 oz.

Oils and Fats

Oils and fats are an important aspect of your keto diet. Contrary to what we know before now, you need lots of oils and fats. You need high quality monounsaturated and saturated fats, as well as polyunsaturated fats rich in omega-3s and omega-9s.

For Oils and Fats

1 Serving = approximately 45 calories

These include:

- ➢ Butter: 1 tsp.
- ➢ Mustard
- ➢ High-oleic safflower oil: 1 tsp.
- ➢ Mayonnaise, unsweetened (made from olive oil, avocado, or grapeseed): 1 tbsp.
- ➢ Coconut spread: 1.5 tsp.
- ➢ Coconut milk
- ➢ Canned & Regular: 1.5 tbsp.
- ➢ Canned & Light: 3 tbsp.
- ➢ Avocado oil: 1 tsp.

GETTING STARTED

- High-oleic sunflower oil: 1 tsp.
- Grapeseed oil: 1 tsp.
- Medium-chain triglyceride oil: 1 tsp.
- Medium-chain triglyceride powder: ½ tbsp.
- Olives: 8–10 medium
- Cream cheese: 1 tbsp.
- Ghee/clarified butter: 1 tsp.
- Flaxseed oil: 1 tsp.
- Coconut oil: 1 tsp.
- Sesame oil: 1 tsp.
- Olive oil, extra virgin: 1 tsp.
- Canola: 1 tsp.
- Sour cream: 2 tbsp.
- Avocado: 2 tbsp.
- Cream: 1 tsp.
- Salsa

Nuts and Seeds

Nuts and seeds are crucial to your ketogenic lifestyle. However, not all nuts and seeds work in the same way. You have to pick lower carb nuts or use higher carb nuts sparingly. Generally, nuts like brazil nuts, pecans, macadamia nuts contain lower carbs, while nuts like pistachios and cashews contain higher carbs. Also, nuts like almonds, walnuts, pine, peanut, and hazelnuts fall somewhere in the middle.

For Nuts and Seeds:

1 Serving = approximately 45 calories

This includes:

- Hemp seeds: 2 tsp.
- Almond butter: 1 ½ tsp.
- Flaxseed, ground: 1 ½ tbsp.
- Pumpkin seeds: 1 tbsp.
- Almonds: 6
- Pine nuts: 1 tbsp.
- Chia seeds: 1 tbsp.
- Macadamia: 3
- Pecans: 4 halves
- Sesame seeds: 1 tbsp.
- Tahini: 1 ½ tsp.
- Walnuts: 4 halves
- Soy nuts, roasted: 2 tbsp.

GETTING STARTED

- Brazil: 2
- Sunflower seeds: 1 tbsp.
- Cashew butter: 1 ½ tsp.
- Hazelnuts: 5
- Pistachios: 12
- Coconut, unsweetened, shredded: 1 ½ tbsp.
- Cashews: 6

Condiments, Herbs, and Spices

There's no shortage of ways to flavor your food when sticking to the ketogenic diet. The good thing is that you can have as much as you want as long as you don't overdo it. Also, look out for spices and condiments that contain no additives as well. For herbs, you can have as much as you can stomach sprinkled into your meals. They include:

- Bone broth
- Cacao (powder/nibs)
- Ginger
- Horseradish
- Lemon
- Salsa, unsweetened
- Garlic
- Hot sauce
- Mustard
- Liquid amino acid
- Soy sauce/tamari
- Carob
- Blackstrap molasses
- Flavored extracts (e.g., almond, vanilla)
- All herbs, fresh or dried (including sage, rosemary, thyme, cilantro, dill, basil, chives, mint, oregano, etc.)
- Lime

- Miso
- Fresh and dry spices (including cumin, chili powder, paprika, curry, cardamom, cinnamon, garlic powder, pepper, turmeric, ginger powder, onion powder, etc.)
- Tomato sauce, unsweetened
- Unsweetened vinegar

Beverages

Because you will be having more than regular fats and oil, you will be thirstier all the time. Staying well-hydrated is essential when using the keto diet. I recommend having lots of water throughout the day. Water quenches thirst effectively. You can add a sprinkle of salt to it if you are experiencing the keto flu. However, there are many more beverages you can also enjoy with keto. These include:

- Coffee/espresso: contains zero calories, preferably black without milk or sugar
- Noncaffeinated herbal teas (mint, chamomile, hibiscus, etc.)
- Green tea, rooibos tea (unsweetened)
- Coconut water
- Vegetable juice
- Milk
- Red or white wine

Sweeteners

Some sweeteners contain a high amount of carbs, while some contain no carbs at all. If you make smart choices, you can also use sweeteners on the keto diet. The right sweeteners won't have any impact on your blood sugar and insulin levels or result in weight gain. The sweeteners you can use include:

- Luo Han Guo (monk fruit extract)
- Stevia
- Stevia + erythritol
- Erythritol
- Splenda

Fruits

All fruits are not equal in the keto diet regimen. Fruits like lemon and coconut are great because they are low in carbs, while fruits like bananas and grapes can knock you out of ketosis and should be used only occasionally.

- Coconut
- Lemon
- Cherries
- Plum
- Apple
- Pear
- Orange
- Peach

- Cantaloupe
- Watermelon
- Clementine
- Kiwi
- Mango
- Pineapple

Occasional Indulgence

These include food substances with moderate carbs that can only be used in keto with absolute care. These food substances can knock you out of ketosis if you don't use them properly. They belong primarily to the legumes, fruits, and berries food categories. They include:

1. Legumes

- Vegetarian refried beans
- Homemade bean soups
- Beans (pinto, navy, lima, black-eyed, black, kidney, garbanzo, cannellini, edamame)
- Hummus
- Lentils (French, yellow, green, brown)
- Peas

2. Berries

- Strawberries
- Blackberries
- Cranberries

- Loganberries
- Raspberries
- Blueberries

3. **Fruits**

- Grapes
- Bananas

Foods to Avoid

The keto diet contains a lot of amazing food products, so you must avoid what is written on this list. These food substances contain more carbs than is required by the keto diet, although some of them can serve in other kinds of low-carb diet plans.

Sweeteners and fat sauces: Honey, coconut sugar, maltodextrin, agave nectar, dates, maple syrup, fruit juice concentrate, brown sugar, white sugar, soda, pesto, tomato paste, BBQ sauce, ketchup, jam.

Drinks: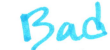

- Smoothies, fruit juice, ice cream, candies, soda, vitamin water, cafe latte, ice tea, energy drink, soft drink, frappuccino, bear, soymilk, milkshake, etc.
- Sugary alcoholic drinks (sweet wines and cocktails); check sugar contents first

GETTING STARTED

- Sugar-free diet foods, high artificial sweeteners, or sugar alcohol like sucralose, acesulfame K, and aspartame

Snacks: M&M's, chocolate bars, donuts, potato chips

Carbohydrates:

- Grains or starches and wheat-based products, like rice, pasta, cereal, etc.
- Most fruits except for limited amounts of berries
- Root vegetables and tubers, like potatoes and carrots
- Low-fat or diet products

Unhealthy fats and foods, including processed vegetable oils and fast food, like pasta, burgers, pizza, etc.

CHAPTER 7
INTERMITTENT FASTING

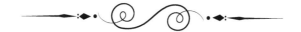

Contrary to what most of us think, intermittent fasting is not a diet but a dieting pattern. It involves skipping meals on purpose, so you choose to eat within a smaller window of the day and skip meals for a larger window of time.

For a lot of people who want to lose weight, simplify their lifestyle, and enhance health, intermittent fasting is their go-to plan. A lot of studies have backed up this dieting pattern, showing that it has powerful positive effects on the body and can help you live longer. Typically, we eat three meals a day, but with intermittent fasting, we can have up to a sixteen-hour fast. Most people prefer using these fasting plans twice a week. There are different fasting patterns:

4. **The 5:2 diet:** In this plan, you will eat 500 to 600 calories on two non-consecutive days in a week but will go back to your regular meal plan every other day.
5. **The Eat-Stop-Eat** plan involves fasting for over 24 hours for one to two days a week. For instance, you might eat dinner today and refrain from eating dinner the next day.
6. **The 16:8 method** is most popular and involves skipping breakfast and eating meals between 1 to 9 p.m., which means you will fast for sixteen hours in between.

BENEFITS OF INTERMITTENT FASTING

When you fast, there will be some changes within your molecular and cellular levels as your body adjusts to bring more access to body fat. Here are some changes you might see:

- Your growth hormone levels might improve, which is beneficial for fat loss and muscle gain.
- Your insulin sensitivity might also improve.
- Cells will initiate cellular repair processes, which remove and digest old and dysfunctional proteins.
- There will be changes in gene function toward protections against disease.

With all of these changes happening at molecular levels, here are the benefits you will witness:

1. **Dynamic weight loss:** Fewer meals mean lower calorie intake. Also, your hormonal levels will change to facilitate the growth of muscles and fat loss. According to some studies, fasting can also enhance your metabolic rate.
2. **Heart health:** When you fast, "bad" LDL cholesterol, inflammatory markers, insulin resistance, blood sugar, and blood triglycerides will reduce, thereby improving your health.
3. **Brain health:** Intermittent fasting also improves the brain hormone BDNF, which leads to the growth of new nerve cells and can help protect you against Alzheimer's disease.
4. **Cancer:** According to some studies, intermittent fasting may also aid cancer prevention.
5. **Anti-aging:** Intermittent fasting has been shown to extend lifespan in animals, although research has not

yet been done on humans.
6. **Insulin resistance:** Through intermittent fasting, you can reduce insulin resistance and lower your blood sugar levels, which protects against type 2 diabetes.

Although research on the benefits of intermittent fasting is still in its early stages, it has been shown to give lots of amazing benefits. You can lose all that belly fat and even enter ketosis faster if you use the intermittent fasting pattern. It's equally more comfortable to manage the intermittent fasting regimen than any other traditional dieting since you save a lot of time finding foods or preparing meals.

KETO AND INTERMITTENT FASTING

It is possible to mix the ketogenic diet and intermittent fasting. This can help you lose more weight in less time and enhance your metabolic weight. Blending these two patterns will also strengthen your ketone production and help the body burn its fat stores more effectively. Combining the ketogenic diet and intermittent fasting is also safe for most people.

However, if you have a history of disordered eating or are pregnant, it's better to stick to the keto diet alone. If you also have some medical conditions, such as heart disease or diabetes, you should speak to your doctor before using this combination.

Bear in mind that intermittent fasting is not necessary to reach ketosis, but it can help you reach ketosis faster. However, not everyone can sustain the two because it might lead to overeating on non-fasting days. A well-rounded keto diet is mostly enough. But if you would like to give intermittent fasting a try, here's a simple strategy you can use:

- 6:00 a.m. – Wake up, drink water and tea/coffee
- 9:00 a.m. – Drink another glass of tea
- 12:00 p.m. – Begin your eating window with lunch recipes
- 3:00 p.m. – Snack a little or avoid it entirely
- 6:00 p.m. – Eat your dinner
- 8:00 p.m. – Eat some dessert, such as nuts or berries, to end your eating window.

Also, on workout days, try using a mid-day workout routine to avoid too much fatigue. This is only a simplified version of combining both. There are many more ways you can connect keto and intermittent fasting for weight loss without having any problems.

CHAPTER 8

Vegetarians On Keto

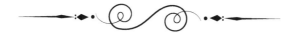

Your vegan diet eschews all animal products, including dairy, eggs, and meats. It's a meal made up of fruits, grains, nuts, vegetables, and seeds. This means you have very little fat and protein and higher amounts of carbohydrates. From the health perspective, some people might be okay if they go on a low-carb diet with some animal products, while others can switch for a high-carb vegan diet.

However, the vegan diet is not for everyone. If you have conditions, such as type 1 diabetes, Parkinson's disease, type 2 diabetes, Alzheimer's disease, or obesity, then you can gain lots of benefits on the ketogenic diet but may not have much from the vegan diet.

However, this doesn't mean you can't still enjoy the ketogenic diet. With careful planning, you can continue your vegetarian lifestyle on keto. This type of ketogenic diet is called the vegan keto diet.

WHAT IS THE VEGAN KETO DIET?

The vegan ketogenic diet is very restrictive, but you can always pull it off and even improve your health. You will consume only plant-based foods, such as fruits, vegetables, and grains, and avoid animal-based foods, like eggs, poultry, and dairy. Generally speaking, your vegan keto diet is a high-fat, low-carb, moderate-protein diet that excludes all animal-based food.

This diet has a lot of amazing benefits, including the fact that a vegan diet can lower your risks of certain cancers, diabetes, and heart disease. It can also reduce your chances of high blood pressure, among many different things. You can also lose weight more rapidly than any other diet plan since you will focus less on animal products.

Generally, you can use these rules:

- Eliminate all meat, seafood, or poultry.
- Avoid all dairy, including eggs, butter, and milk.
- Get rid of animal-based ingredients, like honey and whey protein.
- Limit carb consumption to 35 grams per day or less.
- Eat more low-carb vegetables.
- Let about 25% of your calorie intake come from plant-based protein.
- Avoid all starches and grains, including pasta, bread, and cereal.
- Avoid most sugary drinks, including smoothies, fruit juice, soda, and sweet tea.
- Use supplements if you aren't getting enough.
- Get rid of high-carb vegetables, like potatoes, squash, and beets.
- Get rid of most fruits except smaller portions of berries.
- Avoid high-carb alcoholic beverages.

To see a full list of things you need to avoid, go to chapter six.

Health Concerns for Keto Vegetarians

It is worth knowing that using the keto vegetarian diet is very restrictive. This means you stand a higher chance of becoming deficient on some crucial nutrients, including essential fats, vitamins, minerals, and protein. However, this depends on the kind of keto vegetarian diet you want to follow.

But then it can be too restrictive. A good idea is to check other kinds of vegetarian diets, such as:

1. **Lactovegetarians** avoid seafood, poultry, and meat but eat dairy products, like butter and milk.
2. **Lacto-ovo vegetarians** avoid poultry, seafood, and meat but eat eggs and dairy.
3. **Pescatarians** eat eggs, dairy, and seafood but avoid red meat and poultry.

All these kinds of vegetarian diets will not place you at more significant risks of nutrient deficiencies. But you can also go vegan entirely while substituting most nutrients with supplements. This means looking out for supplements that can provide fat-soluble vitamins like A, D, K2, and B12, iron, calcium, zinc, and long chain fatty acids, like DHA and EPA.

Eating Soy Products on the Vegan Keto Diet

Some researches have shown that soy's estrogen-mimicking molecules may be associated with breast cancer. However, the research on humans tells a different story entirely. Some research on humans shows that soy consumption may reduce the risk of breast cancer in women and prostate cancer in men. So, the impact of soy on health has become a highly debated issue.

However, soy is safe in many instances and can contribute to your general health, whether as a male or female. Most people are okay with it, but a handful of us may also have thyroid issues to contend with after increasing their intake of soy foods.

If you have any hypothyroid symptoms like cold sensitivity, constipation, fatigue, unexplained weight loss, or dry skin after increasing your soy intake, then you can counter such effects by taking goitrogen-containing foods like cruciferous vegetables, such as kale and broccoli, or adding iodine-rich sea vegetables to your meal.

THE SOLUTION

Following the vegan keto diet can be easy if you understand what you can include and things you should avoid. Also, there are lots of healthy food alternatives to some meat-based products, which will help you reap more benefits. Ideally, you should try as much as possible to have only 35 grams of carbohydrates a day and eat plenty of low-carb vegetables.

In addition, let 25% of your calorie intake come from plant-based proteins and 70% of your calorie intake come from plant-based fats. You can also implement strategies, like:

- Use vegan egg replacements.
- Eat fewer fake meats and overly processed soy products.
- Prepare seeds and nuts properly before eating.
- Use plant-based oils, like avocado oil, MCT oil, olive oil, and coconut oil.
- Use iodine-rich foods, like seaweeds.
- Eat more fermented foods, like kimchi, natto, and sauerkraut.
- Use vitamin C-rich foods to boost your iron absorption.

And most importantly, make sure you are having the right amount of carbs, fats, calories, and protein. As a keto beginner, you should also use a keto calculator, so you can understand the numbers you should aim for.

LIMITING CARBS

Naturally, the vegan diet is high-carb based, but when on the vegan keto diet, you must bring those calories down. However, it isn't expected that you eat fewer carbs as you would have done otherwise on the standard ketogenic diet. Those figures are almost impossible to achieve on the vegan keto diet. As specified earlier, you will need to go as low as 35 grams, but it's equally possible to achieve a lot with 50 grams of carbs a day. On the vegan keto diet, you will cut out not only pasta, rice, or bread but nearly all fruits. The only fruits you will have to rely upon include olives, blueberries, coconuts, cranberries, raspberries, tomatoes, watermelon, limes, lemons, avocadoes, and strawberries.

You also have to avoid accessible plant protein sources, like pulses, legumes, buckwheat, and quinoa. This is because they are very high in carbs as well. Aim to have spinach, zucchini, avocado, brussels sprouts, and cauliflower as your ideal low-carb vegetables.

The vegan keto diet also has great alternatives for animal-based products as contained in the table below.

Great Vegan Keto Alternatives

Regular meals	Keto Alternatives
Dairy Foods	
Milk	Almond milk, coconut milk
Cream	Coconut cream
Eggs (for meals)	Veggies, Silken tofu
Eggs (for cooking)	Flaxseed
Butter	Vegan butter/coconut oil
Cheese	Vegan cheese
Grains and Starches	
Tortillas	Flax tortillas

Pasta	Zucchini noodles, shirataki noodles
Sandwich bread	Lettuce wraps
Rice	Cauliflower rice
Oatmeal	Oatmeal (made with protein powder, coconut butter, and coconut flour)
Pancakes	Peanut butter pancakes
Cereal	Flax granola, chia pudding
Mashed potatoes	Cauliflower mashed potatoes
Waffles	Almond flour waffles
Desserts	
Brownies	Almond flour, avocado, and macadamia mixture
Ice cream	Low-carb sorbet, avocado ice cream
Pudding	Avocado pudding
Snacks	
Crackers	Chia seed crackers
Chips	Dehydrated vegetables (such as kale chips)

IDENTIFYING HEALTHY PLANT-BASED PROTEINS

Legumes, grains, and many more plants contain protein, but they are not ideal for keto. That's because they have more carbs in them than protein, making them healthy sources of protein, but due to their higher amount of carbs, they can knock you out of ketosis. However, if you aren't getting a lot of protein, then your body will not function properly, resulting in a lot of adverse effects, such as muscle loss.

You have to get both complete and incomplete proteins. For the complete proteins, only a handful are allowed in the vegan keto diet. They include soybeans, flaxseed, chia, hemp seed, and tofu. You can also have cottage cheese, or peanut or almond butter as well. Every vegetable has some form of protein, although it is incomplete. So, you can still get enough proteins if you vary between the complete and incomplete proteins. Whether you are exercising or not in the vegan ketogenic diet, it's essential to have about 1.2–1.7 g per kg of your body weight in plant-based protein.

GETTING ENOUGH FAT

Your entire diet plan rests on being able to have enough fat in your diet. You can get your saturated fats from palm oil or coconut oil. For polyunsaturated fats, your sources might range from soybeans, tofu, sunflower seeds, walnuts, corn oil, and soybean oil. With regards to monounsaturated fats, your food sources will include nuts and seeds, as well as avocados, avocado oil, sesame oil, canola oil, and olive oil.

However, you must make sure you are getting enough omega-3 and omega-9 fatty acids from the healthy oils and not overdoing it with the omega-6 fatty acids found in many vegetable oils.

Omega-6s are more abundant in nature than the others, but they aren't terrible. You have to make sure they are not higher than omega-3s, as having a high ratio of omega-6 to omega-3 has been linked to cancer, autoimmunity, and health diseases. The ideal way to get enough fat in your plant-based keto diet is by using them for cooking and salad dressings. That way, you can have a lot alongside healthy fat-soluble vitamins, like vitamins A, D, E, and K.

Also, make sure you are enjoying healthy keto fats and condiments as you can see in an earlier chapter as well. Don't forget to increase your variety of herbs and spices, as those are essential in the vegetarian diet. They will provide additional sources of micronutrients without adding a lot of carbs to your diet plan.

USING SUPPLEMENTS ON THE VEGAN KETO DIET

Generally, the vegan keto diet has lots of amazing benefits, but it also has some potential limitations. Vegan diets, especially the vegan keto recipes, lack some critical nutrients if you do not plan properly. However, relying on your meals alone for all the nutrients you need can be difficult. Vitamin D, vitamin B12, zinc, vitamin K2, iron, omega-3 fats, calcium, and many others are some nutrients you might lack in your vegan keto diet. Also, compounds like creatine, taurine, and carnosine aren't found in plant-based foods. Therefore, it's essential to take supplements to make up for these vitamins.

I recommend you use these strategies to boost your meals with supplements:

- Use a vegan supplement form of vitamin D3 (Cholecalciferol).
- Use B vitamin supplements, especially vitamin B12.
- Use a vegan DHA + EPA supplement.
- Eat lots of green leafy vegetables and fermented natto soy to get more vitamin K2.
- Use zinc supplements.
- Add one, two, or all three of these compounds as a supplement: creatine, carnosine, and taurine.

- Boost iron absorption by using vitamin C, but you can also supplement with a heme iron supplement.
- Use vegan protein powders.

CHAPTER 9

YOUR GAME PLAN

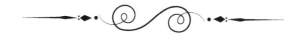

You can follow the keto diet with surprising ease if you develop a game plan. Your game plan will help you visualize what you want to achieve within the next few weeks or months. It's not okay to begin this diet with the mindset of "Let's see what I lose in the first week," or "I'm going to put a little of it in here and see how it works for me."

The keto diet is a long-term plan that requires a better strategy than that. It is not a crash diet where you rapidly lose a lot of weight and gain it back within a few weeks. It is a steady plan that will help you lose weight and ensure that it stays off. I have met a lot of people who have been using the keto plan for many years. But before you build your keto meal plan and establish your goals, it's crucial to develop the right mindset.

The success you will see in this fantastic diet plan begins from your mind. You have to look at yourself positively. You have to stop seeing yourself as a failure. Forget about all those sayings that because you can't get rid of the extra weight, then it's all your fault. Whatever happened before is in the past. You have a new life to create—new habits, new benefits, and growth. Stop thinking in self-destructive terms! The best way to enjoy the keto diet is by looking at those amazing benefits rather than trying to talk down on yourself. Stop stressing over those little "imperfections" people have been pointing out.

Adopt the ketogenic diet not only because you want to lose weight but because you want a better lifestyle. You love yourself, body, and mind. So, you want to fuel it with healthier food sources. Don't think about the weight loss; think about the benefits you will receive. Visualize the youthful skin you will develop in a few months. The ketogenic diet improves your brain function above its regular capacities. Think about the enhanced focus you will have in a few weeks. Every time you enjoy that fat-filled recipe, envision how well you are supercharging your brain and, of course, your body.

The keto lifestyle is all about learning new things—recipes, habits, and eating patterns. You are getting rid of the old and enjoying better habits and, of course, better mental health. When you feel as though you are losing the battle, it's only essential you remember one little fact: You are incredible! So, if you slip, don't panic. A few slip-ups won't ruin your ketogenic regimen. All you have to do is simple: move forward. Reinforce your habits with positive decisions at all times, and ultimately, you will overcome all of those old habits and cravings.

ESTABLISHING YOUR GOALS

As said earlier, you have to be strategic about using the keto diet. It's possible your central focus is to lose weight, but that shouldn't be your entire goal plan. What I mean is that losing weight is a broad term that means a lot of different things to different people. Instead, think in terms of specific, measurable, attainable, realistic, and time-bound (SMART) goals. Ask yourself these questions:

What kind of weight do I want to lose in the next two months?

Do I want to become healthier for the rest of my life?

Do I want to control diabetes?

Do I want to improve my heart health?

Write down your answers and think of more reasons why you want to use the ketogenic diet and what you can do to incorporate the diet slowly into your lifestyle. Some people are quick to cut out sugar intake drastically.

Here are some examples of smart goals you can use:

- I will measure my portion size for the next three months.
- I will drink 60 oz. of water daily.
- I will stop drinking all kinds of sugar-filled drinks.
- I want to limit carbs to 20 grams and lose 4 lbs. in a month.
- I will track my macronutrients for the next two months.

When tired of trying different diets, the only way to move forward is by planning. Make a list of your goals and organize them accordingly. Now, you can start tracking them, and in only a short while, you will see incredible results.

KETO AND EXERCISE

You can also add exercise into your keto diet plan. However, your diet might affect the exercise you need, at least for the first few weeks. It's vital to add exercise to your keto diet plan, although some people do well without it.

However, exercising on the keto diet can help you burn two to three times more calories than you can see in ultra-endurance athletes. Exercising on ketosis can also help you maintain your blood glucose levels, especially in obese individuals. Contrary to expectations, you will perform better when you add exercise to your keto regimen.

For the first few weeks, you may have to avoid intense exercises. This is because the first weeks might be miserable, primarily due to the keto flu. But it's equally possible to adjust your keto diet plan so it accommodates your high-intensity exercise plan. It's also essential when using exercise on keto that you don't eat too little. You can use this rule of thumb: eat 15–30 grams of fat within thirty minutes before your workout and thirty minutes after your workout. This ensures that your muscles have adequate glycogen without leaving ketosis. However, the first week on ketosis is not a good time to use a new workout regimen. That's because you won't feel too great about it. It's often better to allow yourself to adapt to the new diet plan before starting a new workout plan. Or you can begin your new workout plan three weeks before commencing your keto diet.

Nevertheless, make sure you listen to your body, especially in the first few weeks on the keto diet plan. If you feel dizzy, exhausted, or tired while exercising, then you have to stop. The first few weeks may be strenuous, but after a little while, your energy levels will be stable enough to accommodate your high-intensity workout plan.

Using Keto Long Term

Most people are clueless about what to do after they have attained their optimal weight with keto. However, maintaining your weight is more important than the actual weight loss. You can't stumble back to those old eating habits because it will only undo all your hard work. Don't let that happen to you.

Make sure you have plans on how you want to maintain your weight after the keto diet. You must understand that weight loss isn't a short-term affair but a continual commitment on your part. You don't have to keep using your original keto plan. You can build a new diet plan besides keto, but you must maintain your weight through a well-proportioned diet plan. Luckily, keto is one of the most incredible plans you can use for a very long time. A general solution after you have achieved the weight you want is to eat a little more fat and protein without increasing your carb intake. Some people can also add a bit more carbs without causing any new cravings. But you must watch your intake. Overall, avoid using unhealthy food choices as this might spike your blood sugar and send you right back on that journey.

You can also switch from fat loss to muscle building. This isn't technically weight maintenance because you will gain weight, but the new weight will be enhanced muscle mass. To do this, you will need resistance training plans, such as bodyweight conditioning, body pump classes, weight lifting, powerlifting, etc. However, they will also require adding carbs around your workouts and increasing calories through fats and proteins.

Lastly, you can also use low-carb diet plans like Paleo. This diet might include raising your carb intake with extra vegetables by 10 to 20 grams. However, make sure your carb intake is through nutrient-dense and fiber-rich food rather than junk foods. There's no such thing as getting good calories from bad food sources. Whatever direction you want to take, make sure you track your weight. Your new plan might give you a bit more weight, but it shouldn't be more than two pounds. If you gain more than five pounds, then it's possible you are putting on more weight and may have to reduce your food intake.

EATING OUT ON THE KETOGENIC DIET

Contrary to what most people think, it's not hard having keto-friendly meals outside your home. You only need a bit of planning, and it becomes twice as easy. You can have fun with your family, work buddies, or enjoy a weekend brunch out with friends. Being on keto does not mean you have to avoid having the occasional drink or takeout altogether. There are lots of low-carb options you can have and still enjoy yourself. Here are some quick tips you can use:

Plan Ahead

Think about the place you are going to. What kind of menu will be there? When on keto, it's essential you take a quick peek at the menu for that restaurant online. This will help so you don't feel overwhelmed when you get there. Check for sugar-free and delicious keto-friendly options. By evaluating meal choices, you can customize a dish that is perfect for you without feeling overwhelmed.

The Happy Hour

You can enjoy that happy hour even when on keto. Some drinks contain no calories, which you can try. Avoid drinks like tonic, beer, and mixed drinks. Those are packed with sugars, and the beer might also contain gluten, which could be inflammatory to you. Go for drinks like champagne, dry red wine, dry white wine, vodka, gin, or whiskey. These are all keto-friendly options because they are low in carbs.

Eliminate the Starch

Check for starch areas in your meals. Remove the pasta, rice, potato, or bread. Some restaurants can help you swap those areas for something else, such as a salad or extra veggies. If you are ordering a burger or sandwich, some might also swap the buns for lettuce wraps. If they can't exchange it, then make sure you don't eat the unwanted item. Keep an eye for recipes with eggs, such as steaks and eggs, omelets, scrambled eggs, etc. You can ask for extra butter or olive oil or vinegar dressing. If they don't have olive oil, they might have a cheaper vegetable oil, which is not suitable for you, so you have to avoid those.

Make Sure the Condiments and Sauces Are Friendly

Most sauces served at restaurants contain mostly fat, which is good for you. However, ketchup is not ideal since it contains carbs. Gravies can be excellent, but you have to ask about the ingredients of the sauce, so you know when to avoid things like starchy thickeners, flour, or sugar. Also, eliminate desserts from your dish. It's better to enjoy a cup of tea or coffee while others finish their meal If you are still a bit hungry, then you can look toward snack options like cheese or berries and heavy cream.

Work Lunches

Try as much as possible to plan your work lunches.

It's preferable to do so every weekend so you can keep a clean, keto lifestyle. It's also possible to enjoy lunch out with your co-workers if you use the strategies talked about earlier in this section.

Don't Overfill Your Plate

The keto diet does not need too much food at all. Leave enough breathing room on your plate as you would have done at home. If you want to eat many things, then make sure you are eating tiny portions of each dish. Rather than focus on filling yourself with food, enjoy your companions. Take water or tea from time to time and count the seconds between each bite of food. Perhaps, you will feel full in no time and avoid taking the extra portion.

Get the Edge Off

You can enjoy pizza while on keto, as long as you can avoid the crust and settle on the toppings and sauce. Some restaurants also offer crustless options; you can ask about it. But often, such options might be covered with rice flour, which is also high in carbs. Try switching for the traditional options and double with toppings so that you can enjoy the toppings. I recommend using a knife and fork while eating, so you can avoid most of the crust. You can also try making pizza at home. There are lots of keto-friendly pizza recipes you can try.

You can also avoid overeating food outside by snacking

on a fat-loaded meal before leaving home. It will take the edge off your hunger and help you avoid all those tempting starch-based options at the party. The keto diet doesn't restrict you from having fun with friends. There are many more ways you can also enjoy yourself while on a diet. Incorporate these tips into your schedule and have fun any time you want without feeling left out.

CHAPTER 10
TROUBLE SHOOTING GUIDE

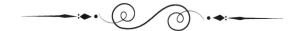

1. Will I lose muscle?

Most people lose muscle initially on a diet, but with sufficient protein intake, higher ketone levels, and muscle-building exercises, you can minimize muscle loss.

2. Can I build muscle on the keto diet?

You can build muscle on the ketogenic diet. However, if you are an athlete, you may have to increase your carb intake above 20 grams.

3. What if I am too weak, tired, or fatigued?

This happens when your body is adapting to the process. It is usual for most people, but you can counter it by lowering your carb intake and using supplements like MCT oil.

4. Do I need a carb reload?

No, you don't. However, some people can do better with higher calorie days now and then.

5. Do I have to eat a lot of protein?

No, you mustn't increase your protein intake. The focus is on the fat increase and not protein levels, as too much protein can spike insulin levels and lower ketones. The maximum calorie amount from protein is 35%.

6. My urine or breath smells fruity. Why is this?

Due to the ketones produced in your body, you might have these effects because your body is expelling ketones through your breath and urine. Don't be alarmed; they are perfectly normal.

7. Is ketosis dangerous?

No, it isn't. It's a natural process that happens occasionally, but in the ketogenic diet, you are forcing your body to rely on that pathway. It is safe in most people. You shouldn't mistake ketosis with ketoacidosis. Ketoacidosis is a dangerous effect resulting from diabetes complications.

8. Why do I have digestion issues?

You might have diarrhea or constipation within the first three to four weeks. It usually fades after that period. If it continues, then you need higher fiber veggies or magnesium supplements.

9. After reaching my optimum weight, what should I do?

Don't slow down or slide back into old habits. You don't have to keep eating keto, but you must have a healthy balanced meal plan. For many people, you can continue with keto with only a little more food.

10. Isn't keto a fad diet?

No, it isn't. The ketogenic diet has been backed by over 150 years of research, which means it has been proven over time to be effective.

Conclusion

Congratulations on joining me on this journey to discover the keto plan. I believe you have everything you need to create a ketogenic diet plan and begin your way toward better health on all levels.

The keto diet is a diet you can find sustainable over a long period. Now, you can begin enjoying your newfound regimen and watch your body turn around for the better. But bear in mind that you won't see results overnight after the first week's loss of water. Your weight loss will rapidly reduce, but in as little as two months, you will start seeing more loss of weight than ever before.

Whatever you desire related to weight loss and aging, the keto diet can help you meet them, while bestowing on you many more benefits as outlined in this book. But you must learn to give yourself a break. You don't have to follow the standard ketogenic diet or any other type rigidly. None of those plans are compulsory. You can personalize it to your own lifestyle needs.

The benefits of indulging in a keto diet are too numerous for you not to try it. Give it a shot, and watch your health soar!

References

https://www.diabetes.co.u

https://www.health.com/weight-loss/keto-diet-types

https://www.healthline.com/nutrition/ketogenic-diet-101

https://www.ruled.me/comprehensive-guide-vegan-ketogenic-diet/

https://goop.com/wellness/health/the-plant-based-ketogenic-diet/

https://www.dietdoctor.com/low-carb/how-to-eat-more-fat

https://www.dietdoctor.com/low-carb/keto/drinks

https://ketogenicvegandiet.com/vegan-keto-supplements/

https://www.healthline.com/nutrition/vegan-keto-diet#drawbacks

http://ajcn.nutrition.org/content/82/1/69.abstract

https://www.ncbi.nlm.nih.gov/pubmed/26892521

https://www.medicalnewstoday.com/articles/320848.php

http://www.ncbi.nlm.nih.gov/pmc/articles/PMC3319208/

https://www.ncbi.nlm.nih.gov/pubmed/12679447

http://ajcn.nutrition.org/content/82/1/69.abstract

https://www.ncbi.nlm.nih.gov/pubmed/29105987

https://health.gov/dietaryguidelines/2015/guidelines/chapter-1/a-closer-look-inside-healthy-eating-patterns/

https://www.ncbi.nlm.nih.gov/pubmed/26892521

https://www.ncbi.nlm.nih.gov/pubmed/2405717

https://www.ncbi.nlm.nih.gov/pubmed/3245934

http://www.karger.com/Article/Abstract/212538

https://www.ncbi.nlm.nih.gov/pubmed/26164391

https://www.ruled.me/comprehensive-guide-vegan-ketogenic-diet/

https://www.hsph.harvard.edu/nutritionsource/soy/

https://www.researchgate.net/publication/24023338_American_College_of_Sports_Medicine_position_stand_Nutrition_and_athletic_performance_Med_Sci_Sports_Exerc_2009_41_709_731_101249MSS-0b013e31890eb86

Made in the USA
San Bernardino, CA
24 August 2019